How To Use Food As Your Fuel

HTeBooks

Copyright © 2016

Disclaimer

This book is designed to provide condensed information. It is not intended to reprint all the information that is otherwise available, but instead to complement, amplify and supplement other texts. You are urged to read all the available material, learn as much as possible and tailor the information to your individual needs.

Every effort has been made to make this book as complete and as accurate as possible. However, there may be mistakes, both typographical and in content. Therefore, this text should be used only as a general guide and not as the ultimate source of information. The purpose of this book is to educate.

The author or the publisher shall have neither liability nor responsibility to any person or entity with respect to any loss or damage caused, or alleged to have been caused, directly or indirectly, by the information contained in this book.

Table of Contents

How Will This Book Help You?

The purpose of the creation of this book, "How to Use Food for Fuel," is actually very straightforward. The main reason why this book is created is to guide people on how they can use food to fuel their bodies. Humans, just like any living organism, require energy to keep their bodies running. The main way in which they can get their energy is through the food they eat. As you can infer, what a person eats has a huge say on their overall energy reserves.

This said, the first way this book can help you is by teaching you how food can help you gain energy. The human body is a remarkable system in itself, regulated by all kinds of processes to keep it running at a high level. The human body has a specialized and specifically ordered system that allows it to use different kinds of materials coming from food for energy. Knowing the different processes that transforms food into energy gives you a better understanding on how our bodies work and how diets should be done for maximum energy and nutrition.

The second way this book will help you is that it would teach you the basics of energy nutrition. There are three main energy sources for the human body. These are carbohydrates, proteins, and fats. Each of these so-called macronutrients is processed in different ways, providing energy and nourishment for the body on the process. Aside from teaching you the basic process on how these molecules are transformed into usable energy, you'll also learn which foods you can consume to get all these nutrients.

Last but not least, this book will tell you about other nutrients that are critical on the energy-production process. While they don't provide much energy in a caloric sense, some of these nutrients are important to ensure that your energetic functions are functioning like it should be. Vitamins, minerals, and even water play a huge role in sustaining the vitality of the human body, so learning where you can source these nutrients is crucial to attain maximum vitality.

Energy and the Living Organism

"What if we ban the word "healthy food" from our cooking vocabulary? I'm not talking about banning foods that are considered healthy. I'm talking about changing the way we think about food overall."

– Marcus Samuelsson

There are many characteristics that define a living organism. These defining characteristics are present in all levels of life, from single-celled bacteria that are microscopic in size to massive whales that are composed of at least a billion cells. One of these distinct characteristics all living organisms share is metabolism. The process of obtaining energy for various metabolic processes, it is the very basis why living organisms (except those who are capable of self-production of energy such as plants) are required to eat food.

How does one define metabolism? It is a series of chemical transformations that helps in sustaining life. Most of them are catalyzed by enzymes, proteins capable of triggering chemical reactions to proceed at an extremely swift rate. The role of metabolism in the body cannot be understated in both the molecular and systemic levels. The products of metabolism (most notably energy in the form of adenosine triphosphate or ATP) are used for other critical biological processes such as growth, reproduction, and reaction to stimuli. This essentially means that without metabolism, life will definitely cease.

The metabolic process can practically be summed up into two contrasting processes. Catabolic reactions break down large molecules into simpler ones. This is most commonly observed when food materials are digested to release energy and nutrients. Anabolic reactions combine smaller molecules to create bigger ones. One example of an anabolic reaction is the formation of various proteins from individual amino acids. However, one must note that catabolic and anabolic reactions usually take place simultaneously on normal states. This is one underestimated element of the magic inside living bodies.

Depending on how an organism obtains the necessary substrates for metabolism, a living being can be classified either as an autotroph or a heterotroph. An autotroph is capable of producing food from inorganic matter. Because of this, they can essentially do self-sustenance at the right physiological and environmental conditions. Examples of autotrophs include plants, photosynthetic algae/fungi, and photosynthetic bacteria. In contrast, a heterotroph cannot produce its own food. This is why they must procure it from other sources. They usually procure it from other living matter such as plants, animals, and bacteria.

This heterotrophic state is essentially the basis on why animals such as humans are required to eat food. While they have physiologic systems that help them sustain homeostatic functioning for a specific time period without food, relying on such systems is self-destructive in the long run. Eventually, there would be a time when they'll have to find a way to get food. It's as simple as that. It's why heterotrophic organisms of all levels (including humans) have developed complex structures and strategies to get food and stay nourished. Energy acquisition is an essential determinant of survival. It's simply the way of life.

The main thing you must learn in this chapter is that most organisms, including humans, are reliant in food to create energy and other vital nutrients for survival.

What You Need to Know about Food

"I like to eat and I love the diversity of food."

– David Soul

Food is an ever-splendored thing. It can mean different things to different people, and it can stand for meanings that go beyond what it really is. Food can be defined in all kinds of ways, but for the purposes of this book, we'll define food according to what it is in a scientific sense.

Strictly speaking, food is any kind of substance that can be used to provide nutritional nourishment for a living organism. Typically consisting of organic matter, food usually originates from other living material such as plants and animals. Once food is ingested by the body, it is then transformed into various components useful for an organism's survival by the process of metabolism. Energy in the form of ATP is one of the most important byproducts of metabolizing food as it drives other essential bodily functions.

The pursuit of food is one of the biggest triggers of the constant evolution of living organisms. Living things have developed all kinds of structures and strategies to ensure they'll gather enough food to sustain themselves in the everyday struggle of life. These adaptations (together with other forms of adaptation) have caused the flourishing of life and the creation of other life forms. Looking at this perspective, it is easy to say that the pursuit of food is one of the main driving forces of evolution.

The same way that food has triggered the evolution of life in general, it has also triggered the evolution of humans in particular. While humans don't have overwhelmingly powerful adaptations (ex. extreme speed, strength, and sensory acuity), they have a powerful weapon on their arsenal: the brain. The human's strong brain efficiency allowed them to adapt to just about every kind of situation and surmount most obstacles Mother Nature throws at them. In the pursuit of a long-term solution for a sustained food source, civilization as we knew it was created as a byproduct.

Historically, humans obtained their food via the hunting-gathering method. Such a lifestyle made them nomads, a lifestyle that is equal parts risky and energy-consuming. Eventually, humans have discovered that they can cultivate specific plants and animals as a source of food, giving birth to agriculture. Because the need to hunt and gather was significantly reduced, humans began establishing colonies at fixed locations. Freed from the responsibilities of looking for food, humans began to focus on other things such as social order, education, and the like. Little by little, civilization as we know it was created, and it all started when we were able to create a sustainable way to procure food through agriculture.

No matter what happens to the world, the pursuit of food will never cease. Both humans and non-humans are dependent on food to get energy and more, and this need would continue to shape the evolution of life. This awareness makes us see food in a completely different light, and on the long run that might be for the best.

Food is essential for sustaining all forms of life. Food also plays a huge role in determining the fates of all living organisms. More than just being a source of physiological sustenance, food has shaped the growth of human civilization as well.

Carbohydrate: The Primary Energy Source

"The brain needs fuel right away, and carbohydrate is the best source."

– Andrew Weil

The bodies of living organisms are made in such a way that they're able to maintain their energy levels in most situations. While almost every kind of biomolecule can be utilized to provide energy for the body, the most important energy source of them all is carbohydrates. Carbs are considered the best option for a quick, strong dose of energy, and for good reason.

Carbohydrates, as the name would suggest, are compounds that are composed of carbon, hydrogen, and oxygen. Essentially, they are hydrated carbon molecules (meaning they contain water), hence the name "carbo-hydrate". Found in either aldehyde or ketone form, individual carbohydrate molecules can combine together to form complex, biologically active molecules. Carbohydrates are the most abundant form of macromolecule found in living organisms.

The most basic form of the carbohydrate is the monosaccharide. They are usually colorless and water-soluble. At the same time, they have a crystalline structure, a derivative of its uniform molecular structure. By nature, each monosaccharide is composed of anywhere between four to seven molecules of carbon, with six molecules being the most common. These monosaccharides can also link together to create complex sugars such as disaccharides, oligosaccharides, and polysaccharides. The most biologically significant monosaccharide of all is glucose, a well-known substrate in virtually all metabolic pathways in cells. Other biologically significant monosaccharides include ribose, galactose, and fructose.

The main purpose of carbohydrates is to provide energy for living cells. Other than being metabolized to create ATP via aerobic and anaerobic processes, carbohydrates such as glucose can also be utilized for other purposes. Glucose molecules are fused together to create energy storage molecules such as glycogen in animals and amylose in plants. Carbohydrates can be used to create both lipids and proteins. Carbohydrates (ribose and deoxyribose) are also components of both DNA and RNA. They also serve a structural function in some organisms, as in the case of chitin and cellulose.

One of the main characteristic of foods rich in carbohydrates is its sweet taste. This makes carbohydrate-rich foods such as fruits a very fulfilling meal for almost all animals. That might have been an evolutionary adaptation in itself, an affirmation of the high stature of carbohydrates in an organism's health.

Carbohydrates, mainly through glucose, serve as the main energy source for practically all biological entities. Aside from being the cell's main energy source, they are also instrumental for a number of vital physiological functions.

Where to Get Your Carbs

"The more refined the carbohydrates, the greater the effect on our health, weight, and well-being."

– Andrew Weil

Carbohydrates are found in all kinds of forms. Considered as the most common form of biomolecule, you can find it in just about every kind of food. The only conflict left to be resolved would be finding the best sources to achieve optimal health. Here are some of the best carbohydrate sources you can get your hands on. As long as you consume these foods at the right amounts, not only would you have an abundance of energy to last the day, but you can also protect yourself from various kinds of diseases.

Fruits

Fruits and berries are one of the oldest food sources for humans. In many ways, it is still among the most effective ones you can find out there. Fruits have an abundance of natural glucose that's easily assimilated for energy production. Aside from providing a direct shot of energy, fruits and berries also contain a large amount of vitamins and minerals that are essential for keeping our normal body functions running. If you want a direct shot of energy, you can't go wrong with chomping on some fruits.

Whole grains

Grains are known for being stockpiles of carbohydrates. After all, they contain a high concentration of starch that is easily converted into glucose. Whole, unrefined grains are the better choice when shopping for grains such as wheat, oats, and rice. They have high levels of complex carbohydrates that are digested slowly, keeping blood glucose levels stable on the process. At the same time, whole grains have more than their fair share of dietary fiber which aids in digestive efficiency and keeps the intestines clean. Whole grain and products made out of it (ex. breads and pasta) should be included in your shopping list.

Energy bars

The word energy bar can be quite misleading, as most people associate it with candy bars that can be potentially harmful in the long run. When we talk about energy bars, this refers to the ones specifically designed for such a purpose. These bars contain ingredients that are quickly assimilated by the body and yet would not cause side effects such as crashing. The best ones are made out of energy-dense natural foods such as nuts, fruit, and whole grains. They contain a massive dose of carbohydrates, just the right amount of protein, and are low in fat, ideal for providing that shot in the arm when you need it.

While carbohydrates can be found literally everywhere, selecting the right sources is very important. For sustained energy (and health preservation), it's best to go for all-natural food or those made with minimal processing. Carbs are high-octane fuel for our bodies.

Protein: An Unlikely but Effective Power Source

"Calories from protein affect your brain, your appetite control center, so you are more satiated and satisfied."

– Mark Hyman

While protein is known to perform all kinds of tasks for the human body, it is not exactly known to be a source of energy. In fact, unlike carbohydrates and fats, the body does not store protein for deployment as a reserve fuel source. Still, when the need arises, protein can be tapped as an energy source. Furthermore, protein in the form of enzymes plays a critical role in triggering all the necessary reactions for energy production. So, to say that protein is virtually useless for energy production would be both wrong and short-sighted.

The main role of protein for physiologic energetics would be its enzymatic role. Metabolism in both the cellular and systemic levels is highly reliant on enzymes to commence. For example, a glucose molecule cannot be transformed to ATP molecules without the series of enzymes that catalyze both glycolysis and Krebs cycle. Looking at the big picture, without the enzymes produced at the stomach and intestines, we cannot break down carbohydrates, protein, and fats into simpler molecules that make them easier to absorb. Needless to say, proteins in the form of enzymes play a central role in both the creation and use of fuel by all living bodies.

One of the main roles of protein in our bodies is that it's the main component of body tissues. As such, most of the proteins we obtain through our diet get channeled to the building and maintenance of tissues such as muscles. However, during extreme situations, muscles can be tapped as fuel source. When we are on a starved state, or in the middle of extreme endurance exercise, the body taps on protein found in muscles as a source of fuel. Protein can be broken down to its individual amino acids, and these amino acids can be converted into glucose. It is considered as a sacrificial system though, as it causes the breakdown of muscles.

Protein, while it represents roughly only five percent of a human being's fuel needs during normal physiologic states, plays a big role in biological energetics. In the form of enzymes, it is instrumental in converting food into usable fuel. It can also be tapped as an emergency source of glucose during times of stress. While providing fuel is not the main role of protein, it can be one when the situation calls for it.

Protein is not all that important as a source of fuel. Its main importance lies in its ability to trigger the necessary processes for converting fuel into energy. Also, it can serve as an alternative fuel source during strenuous exercise and prolonged fasting.

Where to Get Your Proteins

"I eat a variety of foods like vegetables, fruit, and beef for protein and iron."

– Sasha Cohen

We live in a relatively protein-hungry world. With more people more or less following a carnivorous diet and fitness buffs espousing the merits of a diet rich in protein, getting more of it seems out of the question. In fact, there is an argument that humans in general might be consuming too much protein these days, resulting in diseases such as gout. Still, protein is considered as a vital nutrient for a reason, so you just can't turn away from it totally. This chapter will list some of the best sources of protein you can get your hands on.

Lean meat

The fact that animal protein is still the best out there is inescapable. While it can be argued that full-time vegetarians can get their protein requirements without the help of meat consumption, it's actually trickier to accomplish. The main reason why animal protein is considered superior is because it comes complete with all the amino acids your body needs, including the essential ones. For those keeping score, an essential fatty acid is one that cannot be created by the body, hence the need for it to be supplemented via the diet. Go for leaner cuts of meat as much as possible. At the same time, go for relatively uncommon yet healthy animal protein options such as seafood.

Eggs

This has been considered as a staple meal for aspiring bodybuilders for the longest time. Of course, there's a good reason behind such a habit. The protein found in eggs is considered to be of extremely high quality as it's easily assimilated by the body. At the same time, it is considered to be nutrient-dense, boasting a high amount of protein per unit serving. It also comes with other beneficial nutrients such as minerals, healthy fats, and "good" cholesterol. Unless you are hypertensive, consuming one egg daily is considered healthy.

Beans

Legumes in general are great sources of plant-based protein. However, beans have a special place in the hierarchy of protein sources. Compared to other plants sources, beans are highly concentrated in protein, easily matching those found in some animal sources. Some beans even contain almost all the essential amino acids your body needs. It is estimated that the protein content found in beans approximates that of a steak of equal serving. To cap it off, beans are rich in dietary fiber, which helps in digestion and will keep you feeling full longer.

There are many ways to get protein without compromising your health in other departments. Provided that you consume them at the right amounts, animal sources are still your best source of dietary protein. Plant sources are also great alternatives as they bring unique health benefits to the table as well.

Fats: Your Power Repository

"Increase your consumption of healthful fats."

– David Perlmutter

Fats have garnered a negative rap over the past years because of their role in modern health problems such as obesity and cardiovascular disease. However, fats should never be taken out of our diet because of these reasons. Remember that fats do play a huge role in our bodies, and the diseases we get from them are diseases linked to excess. To get a better idea of why we should never shy away from fat, you must learn first its value in bodily functions.

The main role of fat in our bodies is that it serves as a repository of fuel for the body. Fat in the form of triglycerides is considered as the most concentrated form of fuel in the body. To put into perspective, each gram of fat can generate nine calories. This is a significant leap compared to carbohydrates and proteins that can generate four calories per gram each. When fat is broken down, it can provide a serious amount of energy. In fact, if all the fat stored in a typical human's body is tapped for energy, it's actually good for at least 100,000 calories!

Aside from being a highly concentrated storage form of energy, fats are also ideal storage molecules because they occupy minimal mass inside the body. Unlike glycogen, fats don't have to be stored with water, significantly cutting the potential weight and space the body would carry. At the same time, excess calories are easily converted into fat through relatively uncomplicated processes with minimal energy expenditure.

There are four main sites in the body wherein fats are available. The most common way it is stored is through adipose tissue. Found in different parts of the body such as the skin, adipose cells are specifically designed for storing fat. It can also be found in the blood in the form of free serum triglycerides. Another repository of fat would be in the muscles, immediately being tapped into once muscle glycogen becomes depleted.

Perhaps the only downside of using fat for energy is that it takes a lot of oxygen to actually decompose fat into forms that can be used as body fuel. It's actually the reason why aerobic exercise is considered the best method for burning off excess fat. Also, because of the relative difficulty of the process for using fat as fuel, it's mainly considered as an energy source secondary to carbohydrates. Still, fats are tailor-made for their purpose: as a high-powered reserve energy source.

Fats are considered as the reserve fuel source of humans and other animals. Often utilized when the body's reserve carbohydrates (free glucose + glycogen) are depleted, fat generates the highest amount of energy per unit gram among all fuel biomolecules.

Where to Get Your Fats

"Even though we're dramatic, we move our faces, we eat higher fat foods, we're the ones with fewer wrinkles. It makes you wonder."

– Salma Hayek

Now that you know that fats are not bad as long as they are not present in excess, it would be vital to also know where you can get your daily fix of fats. Not all fat sources are made equal. For example, some are abundant on carcinogenic trans fats while others are abundant in saturated fats that are potentially destructive to your cardiovascular system. Just as important as regulating your daily fat consumption, it would also be a great idea to qualify which foods you would be relying on as a fat source. This list consists of some of the best sources of healthy fats you can consume daily.

Fish

Certain fishes, particularly those that thrive in deep sea waters, have meats with a high amount of fat. While some dieters may pause upon hearing this, fishes such as tuna, sardines, mackerel, and salmon are among the healthiest sources of fat around. They have an abundance of omega-3 fatty acids that promote the healthy functioning of both nervous and cardiovascular systems. It also helps in reducing the effects of inflammatory diseases such as rheumatoid arthritis. What's more, fish is a great source of protein and other nutrients.

Avocado

This is one of the deceptively great sources of fats out there. There used to be a time when people were shying away from consuming avocados because of their egregiously high concentration of fat (a medium-sized avocado contains around 30 grams of fat!). However, more nutritionists are now recommending the consumption of avocados because most of its fat content is composed of healthy monounsaturated fats. Such fats are directly linked to lowering bad cholesterol levels in the blood. As long as it's consumed in regulation, there's no reason why you can't enjoy an avocado or two.

Olive oil

This is considered as one of the most premium forms of edible oil for a reason. This Mediterranean staple is considered perhaps the healthiest form of vegetable oil around. One reason why it's considered to be healthy is because of its high concentration of monounsaturated fatty acids that lower bad cholesterol levels in the blood without resorting to medications. In fact, 80 percent of this oil's fat content is of the unsaturated kind, mainly oleic acid. Olive oil is highly regarded to be cardioprotective, increasing HDL levels while reducing the risk of atherosclerosis.

It is not just about how much fat you ingest in a day, but it is also about what kinds of fat you ingest. While the fact that your daily fat consumption should always be regulated, you are best served to eat higher servings of good cholesterol and unsaturated fats.

Other Nutrients Important for Body Energetics

"It's better to get the nutrients you need from food, not supplements."

– Gail Simmons

Macronutrients such as carbohydrates, fats, and proteins can provide the raw ingredients necessary to produce energy. However, it is not enough that you have a fuel source to create energy. You also need to have other components to ensure that your energy production processes operate like they should. Just like in a machine, other additives either initiate or amplify the process of burning fuel. Here are some nutrients you must consume to keep your energy levels up.

Vitamin C

This vitamin, also known as ascorbic acid, is better known for its role in boosting immunity and as an antioxidant. What most people don't know about Vitamin C is that it also plays a huge role in bioenergetics. This is because it helps in maintaining the health of the adrenal glands, a crucial part of the energy production pathways in humans. Also, it helps with iron absorption (more on the role of iron later). Malaise and lethargy, two symptoms associated with the Vitamin C deficiency disease scurvy, are proof of this vitamin's role in energy production.

Iron

This mineral plays a massive role in ensuring that the body has enough energy to last the day. This mainly stems for iron's role in the chemical structure of hemoglobin, the protein that binds oxygen into the blood. If there is not enough iron, it results in anemia, a condition where there's either not enough red blood cells or hemoglobin. One of the presentations of anemia is general weakness because the patient experiences lack of oxygen circulation. Have enough iron in your system, get enough oxygen circulation in your system, and you'll feel significantly livelier almost right away.

Magnesium

This is another mineral that you must consume for increased energy reserves. The effects of magnesium in our bodies with regards to energy consumption are twofold. First, it is considered as one of the factors needed to make the cellular metabolic pathways proceed. Hence, without enough magnesium, you cannot create enough ATP. Also, magnesium is well-known for inducing rest. It aids in the relaxation of muscles and also induces sleep. All in all, magnesium fuels us by triggering our metabolism and helping us rest.

Potassium

This mineral is one of the best minerals for instantaneously boosting our energy. Potassium plays a very important role in muscle contraction. Once muscle cells run out of potassium, they aren't able to contract like they use to, either resulting to increased weakness or a higher propensity of cramps. Other than this, potassium also has a big role in maintaining proper water balance and a normal heart rate. Squash and bananas are among the best sources for this all-important mineral.

B Vitamins

All the B vitamins play a vital role in energy metabolism. While these vitamins share a common name, each is actually chemically distinct from one another. However, it was observed that most of these vitamins are found on the same foods and all play a role in converting fuel from food and storage molecules into energy. A deficiency in any of these nutrients would result to generalized weakness. There's a good reason why B vitamins are always included as an ingredient in all energy boosting products.

It is not enough that you get enough macronutrients into your system for fuel. You'll also need micronutrients such as vitamins and minerals to ensure all that fuel would be converted into usable energy.

A Sampling of the Best Energy Foods

"I like to take care of myself and know what foods I should be eating."

— Doutzen Kroes

A number of foods have already been mentioned in different parts of this book to be specifically helpful in promoting energy production. Still, I find it potentially helpful if I can include some more foods that you can add to your diet to significantly boost your energy levels. These foods, combined with healthy habits, can take your energy up another notch and make you more effective in your everyday tasks.

Spinach

Remember how Popeye became super powerful when he was able to eat his spinach? As it turns out, there is actual scientific basis on the secret weapon of one of the greatest characters of the cartoon world. Spinach is rich in magnesium, a nutrient that relaxes the muscles and catalyzes energy production. The combination of pumped up muscles and available energy translates to explosive muscular performance, an indicator of superior energy.

Banana

This is one fruit that you must not leave out from your food list. Just like most fruits, it has an abundance of glucose that translates to an instantaneous energy boost. Beyond this, it also contains vitamins that help in the body's immune function. It's also one of the best natural sources of potassium, which is vital for maintaining muscular and cellular function. A banana for dessert is great fuel for the day.

Melon

Melons are one of the most underrated energy-giving foods out there. Whether it's a watermelon, a honeydew, or a cantaloupe, melons are packed with a lot of energy-giving nutrients. Aside from having a good amount of vitamins and minerals per serving, they also contain a lot of water. Keeping yourself hydrated is one of the best ways to preserve your energy. In fact, studies have shown that preventing water loss is one of the best ways to sustain energy.

Oats

This is one grain that stands out when it comes to providing your body with enough fuel. First, it is mainly composed of complex carbohydrates that are digested slowly. This prevents the flooding of glucose in the bloodstream (one cause of energy swings) and also ensures that there's a sustained flow of glucose in the bloodstream for longer periods, which regulates irregular hunger cycles that affect energy. Also, its abundance of dietary fiber allows for prolonged digestion, ensuring efficient breakdown and absorption of nutrients.

Food should always be your main source of fuel. Choosing the right stuff would be the first step towards ensuring peak physical performance. By including these foods in your diet, you can be assured of sustained energy throughout the day.

How to Apply Key Ideas for the Best Results?

For humans, food is and will always be the fuel for our bodies. Hence, it can be said that the food we eat would provide the fuel we need to accomplish everything that we need to do in order to strive and thrive. That said, what we need to do to ensure that our bodies would always be in peak condition is straightforward: it all starts with the food we eat. Here are some of the key ideas you must apply to get the best results.

Have enough carbohydrates

Carbohydrates are your primary source of energy. As they are easily transported in the bloodstream and assimilated by your cells, carbs can instantly fuel your body. Simple carbohydrates are great for an immediate energy boost, while complex carbohydrates are great for ensuring you have enough energy for the entire day. A steady mix of fruit and whole grains is all you need for a healthy dose of carbohydrates.

Have enough proteins

Proteins are not considered to be a primary source of fuel, but they do play a major role in keeping your energy up. First, proteins can be tapped as an emergency fuel source during times of starvation. Second, proteins in the form of enzymes play a critical role in keeping your metabolic processes running. Get your protein fix through both plant and animal sources.

Have enough fats

While they are maligned by many, fats do have strategic importance in bioenergetics. As the primary storage source of energy for the body, they are extremely valuable for sustaining our bodies during prolonged activity and fasting. Also, fats are the most energy-dense fuel for our bodies. As long as they are consumed in moderation, healthy fat sources are critical in maintaining a healthy body.

Have enough vitamins and minerals in your diet

Vitamins and minerals, while they are not directly utilized by the body as fuel, play a crucial role in ensuring vital body functions stay running. Have enough doses of them and your body will run like a well-oiled machine all the time. Both plant and animal food sources will provide you the necessary vitamins and minerals you need. The key to getting all these nutrients is to keep your diet balanced.

Keep your body in shape

Beyond eating the right food for fuel, there are many ways to ensure your body will perform at the highest level. Getting enough rest and sleep would ensure that your body will recuperate from the wear and tear of daily activities. Getting enough exercise keeps your body systems in top shape. Last but not least, avoiding stress and other stressful agents would greatly help in maintaining your physical vitality.

www.ingramcontent.com/pod-product-compliance
Lightning Source LLC
Chambersburg PA
CBHW060107300526
45787CB00018B/1784